In My Misfortune, I Am Most Fortunate

TERESA RENDA CARLSON

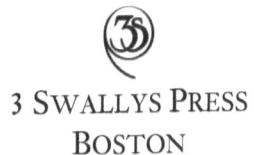

3 SWALLYS PRESS
BOSTON

Copyright © 2021 by Teresa Renda Carlson
Cover design by Pam Germer
All rights reserved

Paperback ISBN 978-0-9987651-5-0

1. Memoir. 2. Body, Mind & Spirit

To the medical profession, which saved my life numerous times and still continues to do so. With thankfulness to all of them, both in Toronto and the USA.

Contents

Acknowledgments	1
1. The Ordeal	3
2. Homecoming	11
3. Pre-Christmas Trip to Toronto	29
4. Christmas	35
5. A New Baby	42
6. An Unexpected New Problem	47
7. To Europe with a Knapsack	52
8. Capistrano, Visiting My Aunts and Gyongyi's Story	60
9. Trip to Montreal Before My Wedding	72

Acknowledgments

Many thanks to my husband Thomas Carlson for his patience and dedication to my project as the Editor in Chief. To my Licia, who despite her busy life always has time to discuss my work. To Nivi, who sees the project through: managing the cover design, choosing the pictures and the layout. A gift to me for which I am forever grateful.

1

The Ordeal

Recently, I was in the intensive care unit at Mass General Hospital in downtown Boston for heart failure, and one of the assisting physicians came to tell me that he would be leaving for California the next day. I felt sorry to lose him, for he was very thorough and good. Reviewing my chart, he was amazed that so much had happened to one individual. "Unusual! The medical language would call you an 'interesting' patient." He asked me to give him a sentence or phrase he could take with him. Without thinking, I said:

"Fortunate in my misfortunes."

I am fortunate to have met my Thomas; our love was and continues to be our anchor, which helped us to stay focused, despite the tenacity and strength of my illnesses. Our idyllic love covered Thomas's first two years in the Army, as evidenced by the voluminous letters exchanged, sometimes twice a day, and became our anchor and daily sustenance. Our glamorous wedding in Toronto, bringing two different worlds together, led us to Fort Knox, Kentucky, where my beloved did basic training. We became very involved with army life; I, teaching English grammar to the soldiers returning from Vietnam; Thomas becoming a Specialist 5 in a platoon where he was able to give the Army a human face by not yelling or swearing, and involving the soldiers in a dialogue where they felt comfortable disclosing their fears and apprehensions of combat in a country foreign to them, Vietnam. Once more, I was caught in the vortex of war. But, notwithstanding the chaos around us, we had our little home in Elizabethtown, and managed to find refuge on the weekends at the Trappist monastery near Bardstown. What peace reigned there; only the murmur of a large river at the foot of the ascent and the voice of the monks singing Gregorian chants in the chapel, which visitors could access from the balcony. The monks followed a strict discipline between work and prayer. They made tasty jams, crusty bread, cheeses and herbal liqueurs that they sold in their little store. We would also sometimes visit a replica of Lincoln's early boyhood home, a one-room wooden structure where an old African American man sat on the doorstep holding an old plate for donations. It is there that Lincoln saw the shackled slaves pass by; perhaps taken to market to be sold or exchanged for others. What cruelty the young Lincoln must have witnessed on the laborious ascent.

How much cruelty was interwoven into the web of life, which calls us to reflect on the purpose of our life. William Shakespeare, in his masterpiece *Hamlet*, expresses this same concept in a soliloquy which begins: "What piece of work is man…"

I was, in the not-too-distant future, to question the purpose of my life, when our idyllic love would be put to a test of endurance, which still continues fifty years later. The enlightening discussions on philosophy, literature and our love of music diminished as we shifted into SURVIVAL MODE: a continuum of medical interventions, laboratory tests, radiation, angst and terror. But fortunately, eighteen months before our chaos ensued, we were blessed with a beautiful daughter who brought us immense joy. She was raised by a loving extended family who nurtured her to withstand the storms that followed. She began playing the violin at age four by the Suzuki method, very popular in the mid-seventies.

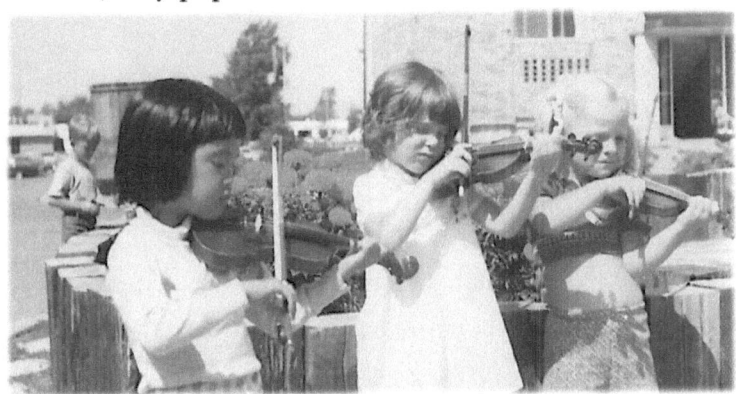

Licia (middle) at Suzuki camp in Wisconsin

We took her to Wisconsin, where she met the master in a class he taught. We could not be prouder to have a daughter like her: sweet, gentle, beautiful and intelligent. What more could we ask out of life? But there was also the storm that tried to tear us apart with my fear of not surviving to see her second birthday; she was only eighteen months when death first knocked at my door. And, unfortunately, many more tempests loomed around us.

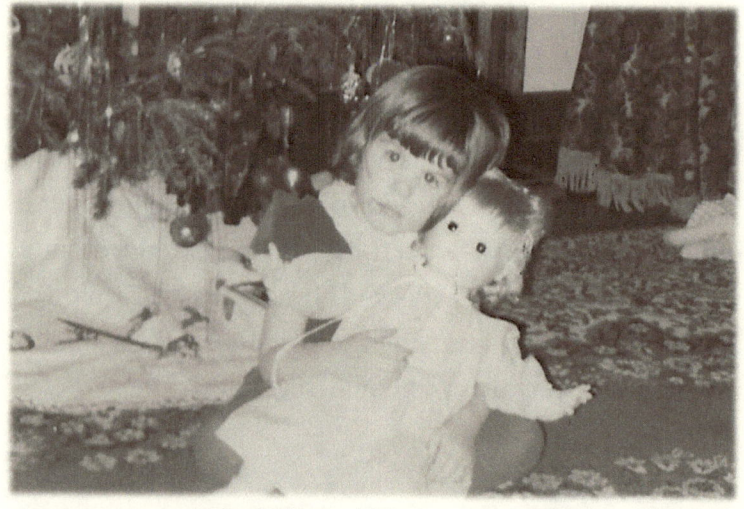

Licia, Christmas 1973, three years old

In the summer of 1976, four years later, I took a trip to Toronto to visit my family by train from Windsor, Ontario. Six-year-old Licia remained with her father, enjoying all the junk food, Coca Cola, hamburgers, Kentucky Fried Chicken and of course french fries, and the Dairy Queen. Thomas was a very affectionate father and entertainer, making Licia laugh, singing, humming music, reading books, going to the Okemos Library, dedicating all day to her. Since the concept of finality permeated my every thought and action, to console myself for leaving Licia behind, I saw my absence as the strengthening of the bond between father and daughter if I stopped living. So I left, seemingly happy, saving all my tears for the train ride, which evoked no comforting sights as we crossed all of southern Ontario.

On my arrival, I saw some of my sisters, who were waiting impatiently and nervously for me, worried about my looks, whether my husband would leave me now, and whether I would survive this horrible disease or succumb to an early death. They, too, were trying hard to obfuscate it all by constructing their own reality: the pathologist was wrong, he misread the lab report, or was given the wrong chart. The large wound stood as testimony to the devastation of a radical mastectomy, for which they thought I was too young. My Gina was shocked by such a devastating wound and immediately called the dressmaker, a friend, to begin working on a wardrobe for me, keeping in mind that I had no right breast. My mother, although unable to withhold her tears, commanded us to go to the kitchen for coffee and cannoli. There the smell of freshly brewed coffee calmed our senses, allowing us to enjoy one another's company, but not for long.

IN MY MISFORTUNE, I AM MOST FORTUNATE

The next morning, during my customary left breast examination, I felt a small nodule. I immediately called the Cancer Center in Toronto, explained the situation and was asked to immediately come in. The oncologist I saw found the lump and did an aspiration procedure developed by the Army to detect metal in wounded Vietnam soldiers. The procedure showed no sign of cancer; nonetheless, the oncologist suggested I see my surgeon. Poor Mother, she was so confused and sad that I had to leave so soon and about the new ordeal. I left on the noon train and arrived in Windsor, where Thomas and my precious Licia were waiting for me. After celebrating my return, our Licia read me a story in perfect French: *Are you my Mother?* which she knew would please me. She detected something was not normal but she went to bed, listening to the voice of her father reading a story. I explained to Thomas our present situation and we decided to see the surgeon the next morning after breakfast.

The surgeon opted for the same procedure: frozen section and radical mastectomy if necessary, suggesting that if I wanted another opinion on a different procedure, he was glad to refer me to another doctor. He informed us that a Dr. Louis Posada would be there at the surgery if I chose. I thought for a few minutes and decided to go through the same procedure. We set the surgery for four o'clock the same day. We arranged for Licia to stay with our neighbors, the Renkoskys, who had four lovely girls whom Licia loved very much. Her favorite book in hand, *Are You My Mother?* accompanied her, plus a beautiful story I wrote for her the night before. We left with a heavy heart, knowing the struggle very well. The lump was benign, but Dr. Posada asked to send two other samples from different parts of the breast. One of them was positive. The mastectomy began, removing some lymph nodes under the arm, which were immediately sent to the lab. Fortunately, they tested negative.

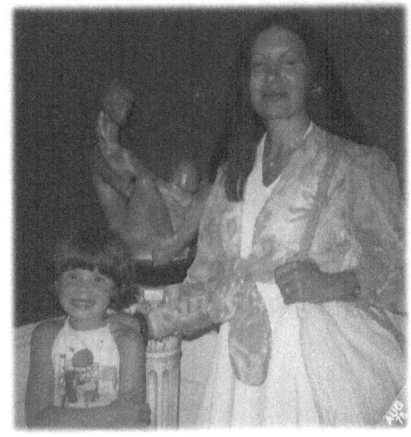

Teresa's birthday with Licia, before trip to hospital for second surgery, 1976

I woke up after the long hours of surgery with excruciating pain but with many of my friends around me. One of them proceeded to lift up her dress, showing me the cesarean scar from the birth of her son. Others were sitting on my bed talking of new decorations they were embarking on. The nurse lost it and asked all of them to leave immediately. I was still howling with pain, the morphine was not effective... pain, excruciating pain. Thomas, desolate at my side, lost for words for the first time in our life together. I sent him home to be with our Licia. A few days later she came to visit me, sad but encouraging me that we would do the climbing exercises on the wall together; she had already sharpened the pencil to mark our progress. After eight days in the hospital, Licia and Thomas took me home, telling me that two surprises were waiting for me.

2

Homecoming

My mother was there waiting with a great meal. Then Licia took me into our bedroom, where there was a pencil hanging on the wall, and all around it illustrations from the story *Are You My Mother?* with the little bright yellow bird, happily chirping. I was touched beyond words and covered our young artist with many kisses for I could not hug her; I was in great pain around the chest, the chest that would make me nauseous to look at when my courageous husband removed the bandage. We were waiting for Thomas's parents on their way from Muskegon a few days after my mother left for Toronto. I felt sorry for my mother, who was suffering immensely, seeing me now flat as a board. I felt like a field that had been tilled and prepared for planting. What would I plant? Pain, anxiety and the fear of death, which had already sprouted and were growing at a frightening speed. Thomas, brave and strong, changed and cleaned the wound, which must have looked awful from the look on his face, which could no longer sustain the masked joviality. I, unable to look at my chest, abandoned myself to the warm waters of the bath while Thomas explained to me that death is like a host that throws a party and asks some people to go into another room, which was equally as pleasant as the first, a thought which did not comfort me. *Un Ballo in Maschera*, the opera by Giuseppe Verdi about the Black Death, came to mind while Thomas worked on my chest; I hummed some arias in my head. I did not want to die, too young, too many things to accomplish and wanting, above all, to see my Licia go to kindergarten.

While I lay on the couch convalescing, my Licia was busy with her friend Stefania, a few years older, the daughter of the soprano Giovanna Colonnelli and her conductor husband, Dennis Burkh. Both girls loved music, especially opera, and decided to write their own opus about a young mother recovering from cancer surgery. First they wrote the story, and then they attempted to clothe it with lyrics, creating some powerful arias. I, lying on the velvet couch along the bay window overlooking the little garden in the courtyard, heard it all. I was moved beyond tears, especially hearing Licia tell Stefania that she would go in to cry with her mother and then continue writing the music on staff paper. Licia bent over me and said that we would cry for a few minutes, and then she would go back to the courtyard, where she and Stefania were working on their opus. Stefania was an excellent pianist, taught by her Nonna Billy, Dennis's mother, who lived with them, and knew how to write the melodies on the music staff. Gregory, Stefania's younger brother, arrived and they made him the conductor and were ready to perform in the semicircular window separating the family room from the dinette. Stefania played the role of the mother and Licia the daughter. Everything was done in a serious way, the girls singing their parts with soprano-like voices; the kids had seen many opera performances under the baton of Stefania's father and performed with ease. The performance was hilarious, opening with a recitative of the mother's wish to publish a book about cancer which she was writing as part of her recovery. The music was played by Stefania on the piano and then incorporated into the performance, a great success. A small reception followed in our dining room, with treats and Kool-Aid. I was touched beyond words, holding back tears with difficulty.

The next month the Michigan Opera Guild put on a performance of *La Traviata*, and I was well enough to participate in the chorus, feeling good to be onstage and united with my friends, especially Lya, wife of Dr. Posada, the neurosurgeon who saved my life. Since some of the artists stayed with members of the Opera Guild, the American soprano Maria Spacagna was with us and we all would congregate at our house for refreshments and biscotti. Licia, Stefania and Gregory were the host and hostesses, loving every minute of it. Gregory serenaded us on the piano, waiting for the girls to sing their opera, but they became too shy to perform in front of the professionals. Lya and her three boys, Juan, Julian and Mitchell, joined us and made us all burst into applause, loving Lya for her musical competence. Richard Voinche, the stage director from New York, was the center of attention for his stage directions, which were innovative and classical at the same time, especially the bed he put onstage during the overture. I lay on it, behind a veil curtain, waiting for the doctor who tried to convince my character Violetta, who knew she was dying, that she would get better. I knew how Violetta, the heroine, felt, as I was lying on a hospital bed weeks earlier listening to my not-so-good prognosis. Perfect for the part, I did not have to act. I was living the real tragedy of incurable diseases. The opera lasted a week of performances and lots of parties. Cancer seemed far away as I watched my Licia's face, adorned with a smile. I enjoyed the moment while it lasted, but tempests seemed never far away from me.

I was unfortunate to be struck with cancer at a fairly young age, still strong and vibrant with a great purpose in life: to see my Licia grow up; yet fortunate that being young, I was able to survive radiation and heal rather quickly from the affront to my body, permitting me to take a trip to Mackinac Island, where we attended the State

Prosecutors Annual Conference. My niece Angela came to help me with Licia, my right arm still not totally healed.

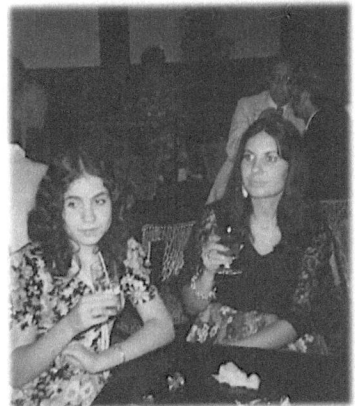
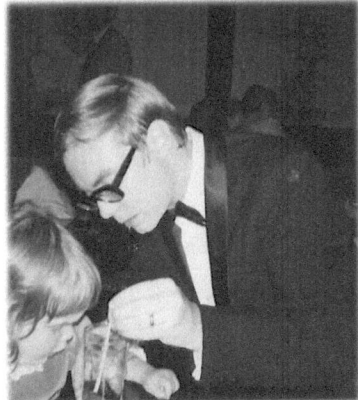
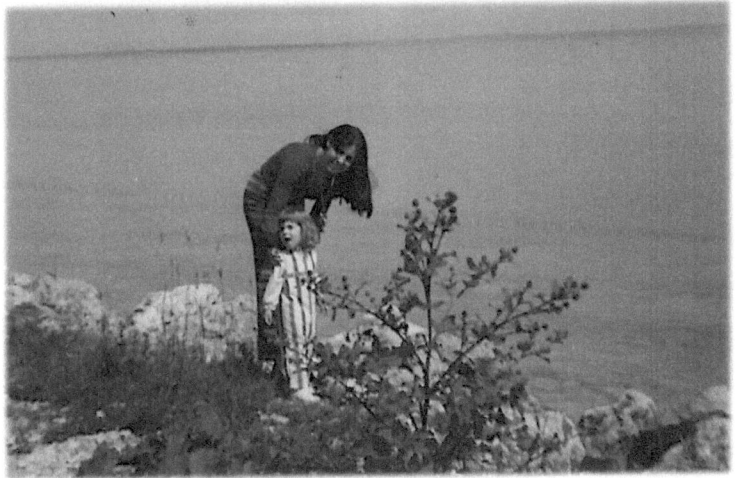

Mackinac Island, August 1972. Top left: Angela and Teresa. Top right: Licia and Tom. Bottom: Teresa and Licia.

We loved the scenery, the horse-drawn carriages (no cars allowed), fudge making and the long bike rides around the island, enjoying the beauty it offered. One afternoon the ladies were invited to a luncheon with Ann Landers as the main speaker, which I attended wearing a light-brown velvet hot pants ensemble. All the attendees clad in long, flowing skirts looked at me disapprovingly, including Ann Landers, who addressed my affront with a short speech on decorum. None of them knew the ordeal that I had gone through, and Miss Morality did not come to comfort me; none of them knew I was celebrating survival from a disease that ravages women's bodies, or the pain I went and was still going through, not to mention the anxiety of each test when death would show its dark cloak over and over again. I learned then to be tolerant of others' actions, for we don't know what motivates them. Life, notwithstanding its diatribes, is worth living, a beautiful gift to mankind.

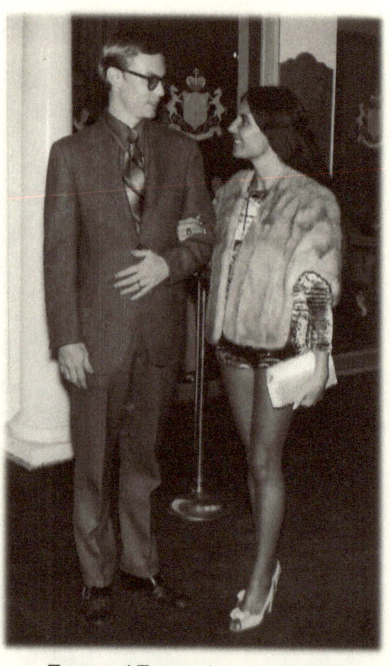

Tom and Teresa in hot pants at convention, three months after surgery

In 2001, during a visit to my mother to reassure her that that I was doing well, I went out to a cafe with my niece Angela and her husband Dominic. Rita, their oldest daughter, went out to say goodbye to her friends, for the next day they were going on vacation. Numerous calls followed, and each time her father insisted that he be called to pick her up whenever she was ready to come home. She informed him that she was getting a ride with a friend. The parents became concerned and decided to drop me off and proceed home. A phone call from Dominic told me to go to their home, for our Rita was in a car accident. I ran into my mother's bedroom, and in a state of shock she uttered: "Povera, Angela! non sa nemmeno pregare" (my poor Angela, she doesn't even know how to pray). I went to Angela's house and her parents were already there, all crying and waling like wounded lions. My sister Nina, Angela's mother (who lived in the same house with my mother), told me that Rita had come to say goodbye to her, and Nina tried to convince her not to go, for Rita was suffering from an eye infection. Rita went upstairs and said goodbye to my mother, who also tried to convince her not to go. After a brief prayer together, she left in a hurry to join her friends at the party. According to the police report, on Dufferin and St. Clair the car, with Rita as a passenger and driven by an older boy from the University of Toronto, who had also been at the party, went too fast down a steep descent, and crashed against an apartment building, where a young lady came out and held our Rita's body in her arms, still breathing, until she died. The boy was already dead. We also learned from the police that it was a souped-up car, unfamiliar to the boy and belonging to his older brother. Our eight-year-old Nina was in bed sleeping, and Dominic, her courageous father, had to wake her up with this sad news. Rita had loved her little sister and had become her little mother, changing and feeding her, and tossing her up in the air like a ball.

At the funeral I had intended to read a poem I had written for our Rita, but I did not have the courage or the strength. A burial followed at a Catholic cemetery where another Rita, her paternal grandmother, was buried. At the burial, with a multitude of people from all over the world who knew and loved our Rita, a picture of the Sermon on the Mount, given by Jesus of Nazareth, flashed through my mind. A reception, Canadian style, followed at the parents' home, with food and loud speaking, which annoyed my mother. She walked home, finding it a sharp contrast to the Capistranese way where people went to the home of the deceased and sat quietly in silent prayer, sipping espresso with biscotti. We arrived home and she immediately went to her kitchen, soft boiled some eggs, and called me, saying: "Come and eat, we have lots of time to mourn our Rita."

September came and Rita's death was still devastating for our family and had sent all of us back into a land of endless pain. The principal and most of the teachers at the school where Angela taught convinced her to go back to the classroom. The children were looking for her and even attempted visiting her at home, the school being on the same block as Angela's. After Rita's death, the young lady who had held Rita in her arms after the crash had been plagued by a constant dream of our Rita begging her to tell her mother that she did not die alone. Angela was constantly blaming herself for not being able to hold her Rita in her arms as she was dying alone. The lady called the police every day, begging them to give her Rita's parents' number, which was withheld from the public because our Rita was still considered a minor, being but a day from her eighteenth birthday. However, the police visited the school, informing Angela of what was happening, and said if she agreed to meet the lady after school, the police would be in the next room if needed. They met and the lady told Angela the details, including the fact that Rita was still breathing when she got there and had died in her arms. The mother was relieved that her daughter did not die alone, and the lady was relieved that she had finally fulfilled Rita's request. The lady stopped dreaming of Rita, although Rita's presence still manifested at her parents' house, with objects from the bookshelf flying around the house, and the heavy sound of shoes like Rita used to make when climbing the stairs to her bedroom.

Because of the strange manifestations, a priest was called in. He went around the house blessing every corner with holy water and a prayer: *Lord, grant Rita rest in your kingdom, and you, Rita, must join our Lord, for you no longer belong here but with God.* The manifestations stopped. I suggested that they move into a new house where they could create a space for Rita, but Nina, her little sister, and her father said that they wanted to remain there, where everything spoke of Rita. They admonished me not to clean Rita's closet or rearrange her room; everything must stay the same, for Rita was still there and everything smelled of her. Both Nina and her dad would go to Rita's closet to smell her. Thanks to the Canadian health system, our family went into therapy free for six months. Nina had a child therapist who asked her in one of the sittings to work on some puzzles, and Nina asked: "What do I care about puzzles, my sister is dead." Upon which the therapist said, let's talk about your sister. No response from Nina. Later when Nina was relating the story to me, she said that the therapist tried to trick her by asking her to badmouth her sister.

Upon arriving home in Michigan, still held by the pain of the loss like a crab holding its prey, I decided to throw myself into creativity. Facing my Zen garden, there stood a wild chestnut tree surrounded by big thorn bushes. With the images of Rita and Nina in my mind, their faces painted white and wearing kimonos from our recent trip to Japan, I began the arduous task of chopping away the bushes and patiently digging out the enormous, deep roots, as if I were digging the pain out of my being. Months later I began to

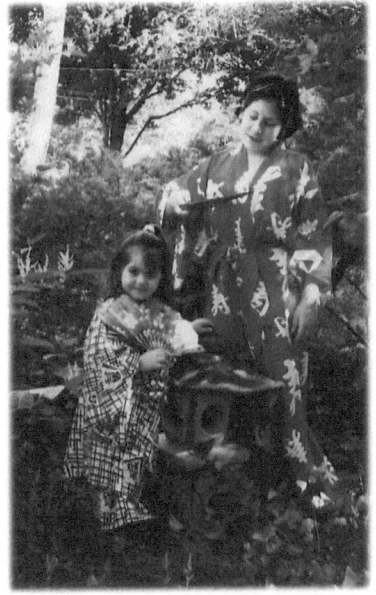

Nina and Rita in the Zen garden

dig a riverbed around the tree, which became a pebble rivulet surrounded by moss, a bonsai, miniature trees and an older bonsai of white pine, standing as sentinel to the entrance of the garden. Two bridges stood at strategic points; the Japanese-style one stood on the thickest part of the pebble dry river and the more conventional one, built by the able hands of my father-in-law, at the garden entrance, where a little pebble lake stood. Bushes of evergreen sheltered the north side, featuring anemones gently moving their long flimsy stems and displaying their delicate white and pink flowers.

On the south side of the tree was a tall pagoda, containing a space to light

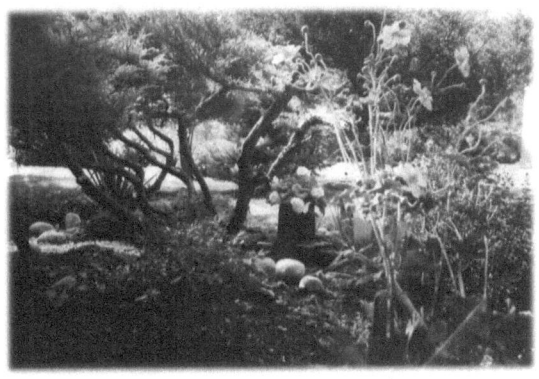

Anemones in Japanese garden

it up at night, and another pagoda, smaller but also holding space for lighting, both near the lake at the entrance of the garden. I was pleased with the garden and its harmony of forms, colors and shapes; a garden that came out spontaneously from my being. I was achieving harmony, inside and out, and was healing.

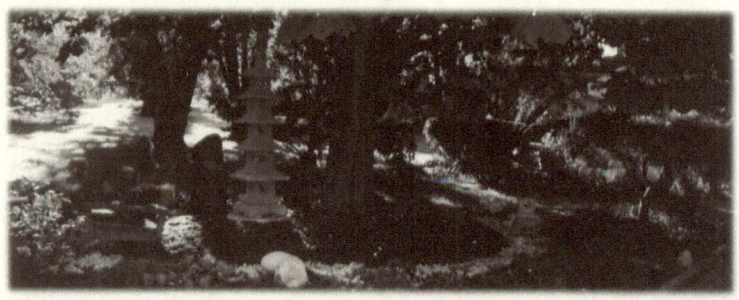

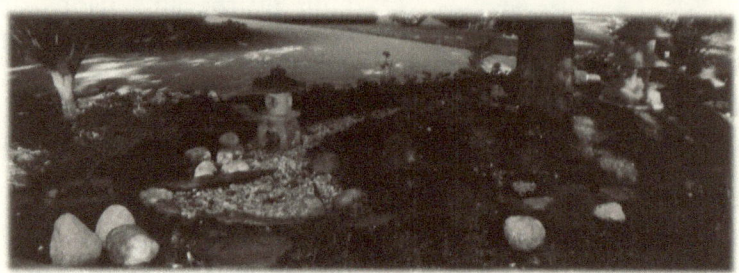

As I sat on the bridge contemplating my creation, Dr. Henry Woodworth, with whom I had written a book called *Needleleaf*, appeared, proposing we write a play about Rita with the garden as the stage. We began brainstorming and started writing every evening after his work at the hospital.

HOMECOMING

The beginning of the play about Rita... and a poem

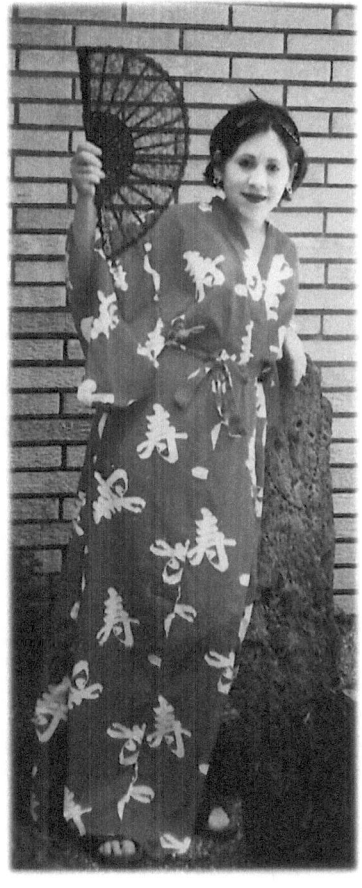

I am a seventeen-year-old named Rita. I am a goddess! Well, I was a goddess... not a real goddess in the true Greek goddess sense, but after I died, I learned I was a real goddess to those who knew and loved me. In fact, my great-aunt first wrote a poem and then a play with her friend, Dr. Henry Woodworth, about me. A sifter is sitting under the chestnut tree in the Japanese garden which my great-aunt built as a catharsis. She is wearing loose-fitting clothes and a red Japanese hat which hides her face but not the sound of the pebbles she is sifting, methodically moving the sifter back and forth, creating a pile of fine sugary sand. The sand which had been dug up by squirrels hiding seeds sticks to the pebbles, muting their brightness and masking their varied hues. The pebbles in the riverbed are not just pebbles, but become drops of water creating a gentle flowing river, which is a mystical bond with all the other rivers joining at the end of their journey to the Greater Sea, where everything becomes one.

Rita becomes one of the immortal gods after death, the goddess of trees. Being in an expansive mood one morning, she began spreading seeds around the gentle river flowing peacefully in its riverbed, singing with the various birds that populated the area. The squirrels were also abundant, chewing the wild chestnuts, but when they saw all the seeds around decided to bury as many as they could to survive the coming winter. The riverbed became heavy with seeds and the earth dug by the squirrels, and the water stopped flowing, the birds stopped singing and the sifter stopped sifting; only mud remained in the river. But soon, through the mud, little green heads began to appear, only to be choked by the parched earth.

Poem about our beloved Rita

>
> We come and go
> Before the night is over
> Like a shooting star.
>
> We feel, we see, we cry
> We leave but a trace
> In the hearts of those who are us

HOMECOMING

Soon we, too, will become a shooting star
Another shooting star.

You look so radiant
Full of life
Not ready for sleep
But what a sleep
You sleep.

Mother and Dad wait for you
They call, they wait, they cry
No, your world is beyond the sky.

We come and go
As quickly as a breeze
Into a night of peace

You are now a star
In the vast firmament
Shine, dear one!
And when night comes
And the world is still
No longer a laughter or a sigh
Your parents' gaze is toward the sky
To see their dear Rita
Twinkle her eye.
Through poetry, my great-aunt tried to deal with her

suffering, perhaps to transcend, if momentarily, her pain. Humans are an odd bunch: they intellectually know they have to leave Mother Earth someday, yet they live as if their stay is permanent; otherwise why would they choose to live within the material confines of their daily worlds, amassing fortunes which entomb them. Believe me, I know what I am talking about; I was once there. Illusions, illusions, we keep weaving them as fast as a spider weaves its web, only to be torn by the housewife's wand. Many people find relief from grief by ending up in front of a psychiatrist who listens and nods, charging an arm and a leg. I speak from experience.

In my youth, too, I landed in one of those chairs because I refused to go to school. I kept telling my parents school was boring, page after page of the addition and subtraction exercises. I quickly figured out that each problem had the same result, which was at the top of the page, except a few that didn't. I put the same result on all of them, knowing I would lose a few points. Well, back to the shrink. I, too, was coaxed into confessing my angst by a white-haired eminent master of the trade who had cracked every nut that landed in his chair. Of course, I assessed him the very first visit and decided to string him along with my silence, while he was convinced that his games and charts would come to his aid. After a few weeks of failure, he stopped the games and the charts and began asking personal questions about my parents and my relationship with them: were they loving toward each other and especially toward me. I wrinkled my brows, giving the appearance that I was using the gray matter encased in my frontal cortex and began to open my mouth ever so slowly... unable to contain his delight, he began to gesticulate with his hands, trying to pull out each word from my mouth, which was expanding ever so wide and wider, only to terminate in a gigantic, feigned yawn.

I did feel sorry for the eminent gentleman and granted him a sentence, and as rapidly as a drop of water tumbles down Niagara Falls, I uttered loudly and clearly: "Did you think I was going to badmouth my parents behind their back?" I left the office with the dear old man standing at the door, a big grin on his face.

Back to my great-aunt and her Japanese garden. The sifter was overwhelmed by the number of squirrels and the sudden transformation of the river into the parched remains of dried-up mud. She had a plan to save the river: She began to dig. She dug furiously, deeper and deeper into the muck, until she reached the riverbed, where water drops gasped quietly, waiting to be released. The sifter knew instinctively the water drops would be there buried by mud, hiding in the earth, needing somewhere to go. Once the first water drop emerged, many began to pour out in bunches, then in larger groups, gurgling out until the space was filled with limpid, bubbling blue water, filling the riverbed, which overflowed onto the river bank, onto the parched earth all around, the sifter's body redolent with pain from the digging, her spirit cleansed from pain.

Our tree goddess continues her journey throughout the earth, thinking of new ways to sow more seeds, perhaps more efficaciously, like seeds resistant to squirrels, or seeds that grow instantly before animals discover them. She continued her mission, a little wiser perhaps, having learned from experience.

3

Pre-Christmas Trip to Toronto

Christmas was approaching and I decided to visit my family in Toronto. My sister Nina was not at the door welcoming me, but lying on the sofa holding against her chest the last picture of Rita taken with her camera at the party, which had survived the crash and was found in her purse. Through teary eyes, Nina told me she would not be living long, the pain consuming her. Besides, she had dreamed about my father telling her he had not seen Rita, which was devastating because the last comforting thought Nina had was that her Rita would be with our father. She chided me again for having brought her back to life during a heart failure at Toronto General when, in intensive care, I was there intently watching the heart monitor. Seeing that it was slowing down considerably and Nina was gasping for breath, I shook her to wake up for her Rita, who would be devastated without her Nonna. She came back and told me she was in a peaceful, dark tunnel, almost ready to reach the light at the end, and then I brought her back. "Why did you bring me back only to see my Rita die?" I remained speechless. She asked me to make some of my biscotti; she liked how thinly I sliced them. I held my Nina's hand for a while and then proceeded upstairs to see my mother, who was watching the Chinese news because she liked the anchorman. My mother did not understand a word the newscaster was saying, but for Italians appearances take precedence over understanding.

I asked Mother how Palmira's twins were and she responded, well how can they grow, they are "children of the plate" (in vitro). Poor mother, technology was not her forte. One day when we were walking down College Street back from the hospital to see Palmira and her twins, we met an old lady from Capistrano who asked how we were doing. My mother explained that her granddaughter Palmira had just had twins but that they were very small, for they were conceived in a plate. The lady was astounded and said, "Today they do it everywhere, even in plates, this I did not know. God help us," and she blessed herself. We walked to the Cafe Siciliano and my mother continued on the subject of the plate. She asked me how they could make love in a plate; she could not comprehend how they knew that. She had always thought Palmira and her Canadian husband were a nice couple, and said maybe it was an ancient Indian custom. Hardly able to contain my laughter, I said I was not aware of the Indian ways, upon

PRE-CHRISTMAS TRIP TO TORONTO

which she chided me for always reading but knowing very little. I excused myself and went to the bathroom on the pretext of washing my hands, having come from the hospital, and I burst out in the most explosive laughs. I came back relieved, bringing my mother a wet paper towel to clean her hands, which she found very cold, asking if I had used hot water. Poor mother, I could do nothing right. We finished our cappuccino and cannoli and went next door to a Chinese art store.

A gentle young Chinese man showed me the latest imports, and my eyes fell upon a Chinese wooden screen, a triptych, with a mountain, cherry blossoms carved on it and birds fluttering around. I decided to buy it for my family for Christmas. While the gentleman was packing it for me to transport on the train, I turned to my mother, who obviously was not pleased, for it was not a Madonna, and said how cute the Chinese gentleman was. She responded with another insult: You worry me, you've lost your *decato* (the sense of measure of people and things). I then informed her we were going to the grocery store, which she loved to visit because she would take food from the bins, candies and fruits, and munch on them on the way out. The manager came and told her stealing was not allowed, to which she responded that she paid for what she takes many times, for she spent all her monthly pension there. Then she asked me why I was buying almonds, don't they have them in the U.S.? I told her Nina had asked me to make my thin biscotti for Christmas. Can't she make her own? She resented any intrusion on our visit; in spite of all the abuse, she wanted me all to herself.

I asked Dominic to take me to Saint Clair Avenue, another Italian hub, where we would find the almonds. We found them at the Pasticceria La Sem owned by Nicolino, the brother of the girls who travelled with us from Naples to Toronto. What a joy to see Gensella there. We talked, bought some exquisite pastries for Nina, my mother and Angela. She kindly sold us some of the almonds they use at the Pasticceria. We went home and Nina was waiting. We began our baking, notwithstanding the lugubrious purpose, and we had a good time together talking about my Licia, our mother, for whom she had little patience, and Angela. Even the twins, who had been her immense joy before Rita's death, were not able to keep her from the wish to pass on. It reminded me of what my father used to tell us: love one another well, for when one finger hurts, the whole hand hurts. I was hurting terribly but I kept my secret; I could not betray her again. Despite the pain, I tried to enjoy being with her, my last time perhaps. The biscotti came out precisely as she wanted, thin, light and with lots of almonds.

The next morning I left to celebrate Christmas with my Licia and Thomas. They met me in Windsor, and we went to Little Italy to buy tiramisu and bread. I was reminded of how we used to make the *presepe* together when Licia was a little girl. She would set the crib and put Baby Jesus in. She loved to place the figurines around the manger, which were beautifully carved by an artist on the Alps and painted with gentle pinks, greens and browns. What a play of shapes and colors interwoven to give an image of Heaven. The faces were fascinating in their expressions. The camels with the three kings were majestic, and the shepherd with a sheep around his neck like a scarf, guiding the others on the moss, which Licia and I would gather from the garden. We would make little trees with evergreen branches and create a little lake by placing a mirror in a little well surrounded by sand. We made small clay houses, creating a little village on the mountains, which were made with sheets of brown paper sprinkled with white flower as snow.

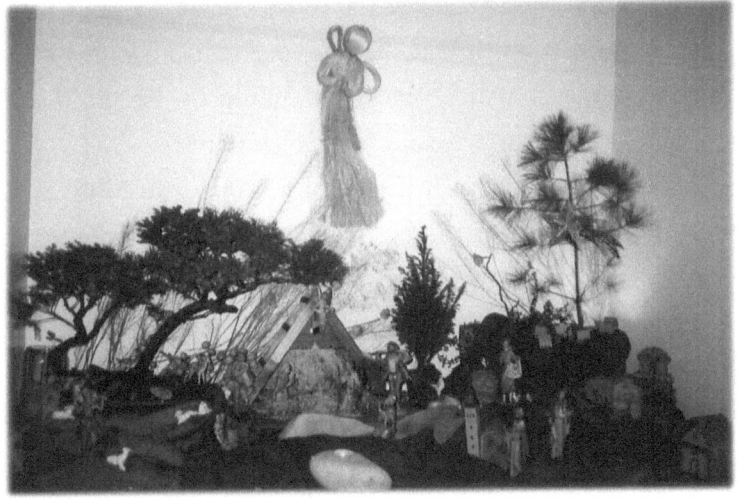

Christmas 1976 *presepe* (nativity scene)

A little town of Bethlehem in our house. Licia would clap with joy and could not wait to show her father our creation.

I heard from my mother that our Nina had died quietly in her sleep, a death very much planned and caused by letting the battery of her pacemaker expire. Thomas came home and together with Licia drove me to the train station in Windsor. My mom was howling like a wounded wolf, and became inconsolable; words ceased to be effective, only silence worked for me. At the funeral home, my mom would go to the coffin often and kiss Nina, telling her she could not live in the house on Montrose without her thundering Renda voice. My poor Angela, another painful burial for her. Our Nina wanted to be buried near her Rita. Our sister Gina was inconsolable too; she had become very close to Nina over the years, depending on her help and advice. It was all unbearable for me to witness.

After Nina's burial in December 2002, the Christmas season was upon us and I decided to hurry home to prepare for a special Christmas after so much suffering, using all the energy that follows a tragic event. I was going to avail myself of every positive nuance, regardless of how unimportant it seemed. We made taralli and pugnolata (small pieces of fried sweet dough adorned with honey and sprinkled with small colored candies).

4

Christmas

My mother joined us from Toronto bringing two suitcases of traditional Christmas food: panettoni, torrone, torroncini (big and small bars of filbert nuts covered with chocolate or white sugar mixture) wrapped in various-colored paper which traditionally were hung on the Christmas tree; torrone al gelato, breads, cheeses, olive oil from Capistrano, olive schiacciate (cured green olives, cracked with a stone and drenched with olive oil), fennel seeds and sprigs of wild oregano from the hills of Capistrano... A feast which brought back my childhood years in that blessed village. On Christmas Eve we fried zippole, a pizza-like dough, for the Christmas supper, which, according to tradition, was comprised of thirteen different foods. After the plentiful supper, we lit the candles and Licia led our procession of three into the family room where the *presepe* was set. Then we went to Midnight Mass, where we also saw a procession to the *presepe*, much bigger than ours. When we returned home, a fellow whom Thomas was helping and had recently been released from prison was in our driveway with two suitcases full of what we later learned were Thomas's suits. He saw us and came to the door holding a Christmas card.

He left and we called the police, who were very gentle so as not to frighten our daughter Licia, or involve her with the investigation. My mother was sad for he had also taken all her money. Our Licia was happy for she got to play investigator, and she exclaimed: "Mr. Smith must have loved me very much, he didn't take my violin, my dolls or my clothes." A sad and disappointing story. We tried to alleviate the situation by eating the panettone, taralli, torrone, etc. All in all, an otherwise good Christmas... surviving the life-threatening tempest and allowing us to still be together. I resumed my teaching and added a children's class in Italian at Licia's school, enjoying myself greatly. Everything was going well.

The Vietnamese Refugee Program was in full force and people were arriving in boats full of refugees to the United States for adoption. We, together with other members of our parish, adopted a family of numerous adults. The family spoke French and only the eldest girl spoke English. I enjoyed speaking with the father in French, who was reticent at first but after assessing us, opened up more. When they invited us for a Sunday lunch, only the older girl and the father sat at the table with us; a little strange, I thought. It was a highly educated family; the father was a diplomat, and they probably went to good schools before the U.S destroyed their land, forcing many to flee. The wealthy ones could buy passages on ships headed for the U.S. But a greater surprise awaited us.

The Vietnam war followed us even in Michigan and would be with us for many years. Around one o'clock one night, Thomas, returning from a case in northern Michigan, arrived and happily announced: "Honey, we have guests." It was 1976 and I had come back from Toronto knowing that I would have to go to the hospital on my birthday. I recited an invocation to God, asking for strength to handle this. And now, a beautiful, young mother, followed by her three children, with one still in the womb, had arrived. But seeing those beautiful faces, my heart melted. The four-year-old was a little Buddha, the way she sat cross-legged. Thomas prepared a warm bath for the children, followed by snacks, soup and sandwiches. We all sat in our dining room and ate; Licetta woke up and joined us. She was happy to have Long, Lynn and Lei to play with. We fixed the beds, two pulled out for Long and Lynn in the guest room with their mother. Lei slept in the double bed with Beh, their mother. Beh went into the bedroom and we heard her chanting, perhaps Buddhist chants. In the meantime, Thomas told me how he had seen her on the highway late at night on his drive home. He got out of the car, seeing four figures huddled together and walking in the dark. At first they were frightened, but after Thomas showed them pictures of Licia and me, they reluctantly got in the car and remained mute like sphinxes for the whole trip. To my delight I discovered Beh spoke French, her father being French, her mother Vietnamese, and that explained her Eurasian look.

The children, after being fed and bathed, went to bed, leaving time for Beh and me to talk on the moonlit balcony overlooking the woods. She told me that her husband was a banker and paid for the boat trip to the U.S for himself and the family. At the dock, he told her that he had forgotten to bring cash with him and ran home to get it. Meanwhile, the boat left and she sailed off alone with the children, sleeping on the top deck for many weeks, in the cold and rain, comforting her children, with Lei, the youngest, only four years old, and another in the womb. I gave her a warm, long embrace as if I, too, had been part of that cargo of frightened humanity, brought about by inhuman political leaders for whom the world was a playground for their war games.

Vietnam had nothing redeeming for its senseless immolation of our American youth, unlike World War II, where I was a living witness to their sacrifice and goodness. If not for the brave American men, southern Italy from Rome down would be populated by Hitler's perfect race:

blue eyes, blond hair and statuesque bodies, the result of the programmed race between German officers and Swedish women. I could easily have ceased to exist, and certainly would not have been able to emigrate to the U.S., marry my Thomas and become an American citizen, which ultimately made me eligible to vote for President Obama and Hilary Clinton. Here were two exemplary politicians and intelligent humanists, a total antithesis of the Mussolinian monster currently leading this beautiful country, to which my Thomas introduced me, and of which I learned to love for its fierce independence and altruism, in spite of its many follies. The first time I saw Trump descending the stairs of one of his fake empires, I announced to the family: "Here is Mussolini incarnate: narcissistic, selfish; watch his measured dictatorial walk, his mode of communicating, creating a false reality, his admiration of other dictators who built their power on lies and fear, vindictive toward those who disagree with him, and creating a climate of fear capable of intimidating Republican congressmen who perhaps would have been more vigilant and altruistic under another leader." Where are the Republicans like Milliken and Romney, Michigan's governors? Thankfully Governor George Romney left us an independent and altruistic son who became governor of Massachusetts, and who provided a health care program for the state, followed by a Republican senatorial win in Utah, becoming the only Republican unafraid to vote to impeach the monster in the White House. He stood alone in a sea of cowardly fellow senators, afraid to open their mouths, except to praise a brute, a cheater par excellence, with a canny ability to create a crisis and then, after the destruction he fomented, promoting himself as the powerful and valiant savior warrior, defying and disregarding the laws of the country and the Constitution, giving himself unwarranted power. A perfect Mussolinian monster, who, ignorant of history, is doomed to repeat it to the end: his demise.

Mussolini would order his Blackshirts to go into towns and villages and exterminate the men they could find and then go to the major centers and announce a benevolent plan to help the widows and the orphans he had created. I was in the piazza in Reggio Calabria, held in the arms of my father, who was beaten every night for refusing to wear the black shirt, the plan being to eliminate him slowly without creating havoc in the town where he was loved by most of the villagers. Many people welcomed Mussolini like a hero who wanted to help the common people, mostly women holding their orphaned babies in their arms. Likewise, Trump deploys in Oregon heavily armored federal militia in unmarked vehicles that whisk away peaceful protesters without identifying themselves and using brutal tactics like placing hoods on their heads to prevent them from seeing where they are being taken. Trump declares victory in his plan to protect his precious monuments of Confederate leaders, which are a testimony to the slavery and brutal treatment of Blacks. Trump is an incarnate Mussolini. God help us.

5

A New Baby

After my second surgery, I returned home and Thomas was handling the family well. How I desired a big family now more than ever. But, back to school for the children. Beh asked me for some warm water and towels, and I went to lie down, still recovering from the second radical mastectomy, which left me flat as a newly tilled field, ready to be planted with the seeds of living. What seeds would I plant? An English, Japanese or Italian garden? I decided to visit Ardis (Renkoski), my neighbor, to forget about my pain.

    I came home from visiting Ardis, and there was Beh sitting with her new baby in her arms, all beautifully dressed in a white silk chemise embroidered in soft pink with silk thread. Lei was sitting like a little Buddha at her side, a picture of serenity and harmony, a divine moment. She offered the baby to me, saying in French, "Elle est à toi" (She is yours). I was speechless and overwhelmed by her generosity. I truly wanted the baby, Lana she named her, but I could not accept her. I thanked her in French and told her that I would help her raise baby Lana but that she belonged to her family. We embraced, a long embrace of friendship.

Thomas and the kids came home to baby Lana, a big surprise for all of them. We did a little homework before a delicious dinner Beh had prepared early that morning before the magical event, the birth of Lana. We had a celebratory supper and Thomas took the kids for ice cream, while Beh attended to baby Lana, breastfeeding in her room, which was clean with no sign of the birth. I asked her what she did with the placenta, and she showed me where she buried it in a hole in the woods behind the house, which she dug herself. What strength; visually frail, but what a courageous young lady in her early- to mid-twenties. I was amazed and became protective of her as her mother in loco parentis.

Beh felt strong and decided to go to Paris to meet her father, who had been a French soldier in Vietnam. I felt it was a little too early to leave the baby, but who was I to teach this heroine anything? She left in mid-August for two weeks.

I had my baby for two weeks, all to myself; Licia was a big sister to the other three; a big family, that's what I wanted. Beh sent us beautiful pictures of her in front of La Tour Eiffel, in a red silk dress, an apparition. The children were delighted to see their mother happy after months of suffering in the open elements. She had prepared them well, chanting

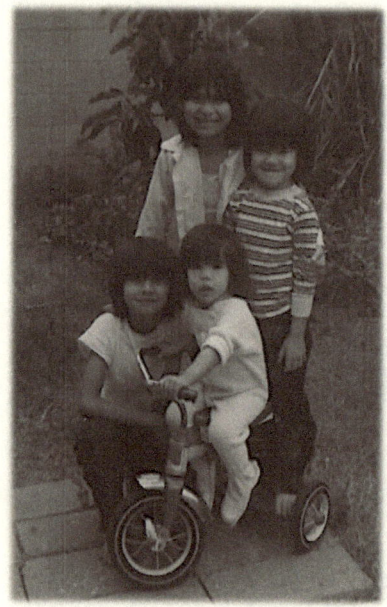

Lynn, Lei, Long and Lana

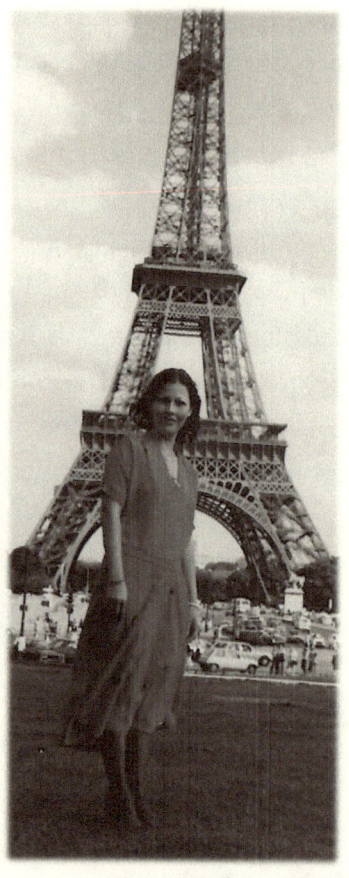

Beh in Paris

to them in their room for hours. What an incredible culture. And we Americans destroyed it for no reason. We should have learned from the French, who saw an unwinnable war and left. The French were allured to Vietnam for the rubber forests which yielded tons and tons of rubber. They denuded the forests and left without providing any compensation for the damage.

Upon her return, Beh announced that she was going to settle down in California, where a large Vietnamese community lived. A sad day in our family. We had gotten used to our new children, but we promised to continue to help her and keep in touch. Our house seemed empty, but thanks to God we had our marvelous Licia, who was growing into a remarkable young girl. A few years of calm ensued and we thrived in the love of one another. *Carmen* was being prepared for the stage and I rejoined the chorus.

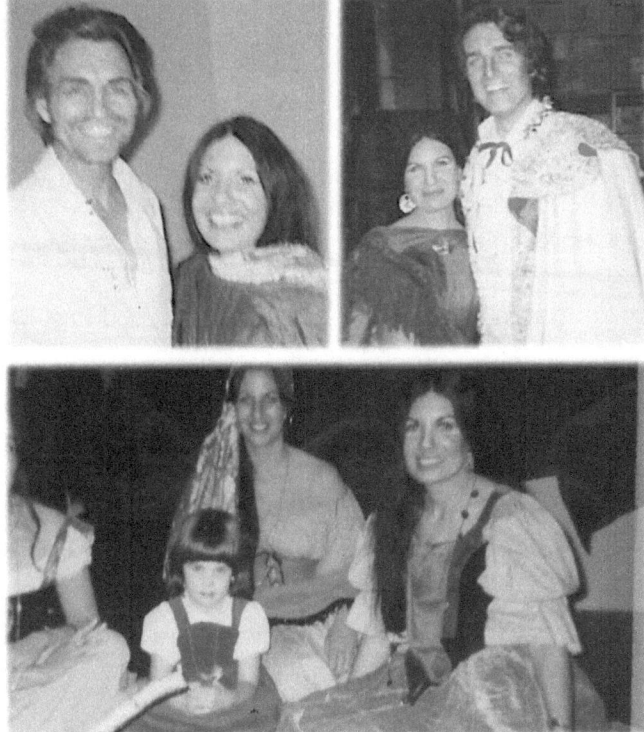

Carmen. Top L: w/ Bill Louis. Top R: w/ Toreador. Bottom: Gypsies with Licia.

Licia was happy to see all those opera singers in our home. She loved people and saw the good effect they had on me.

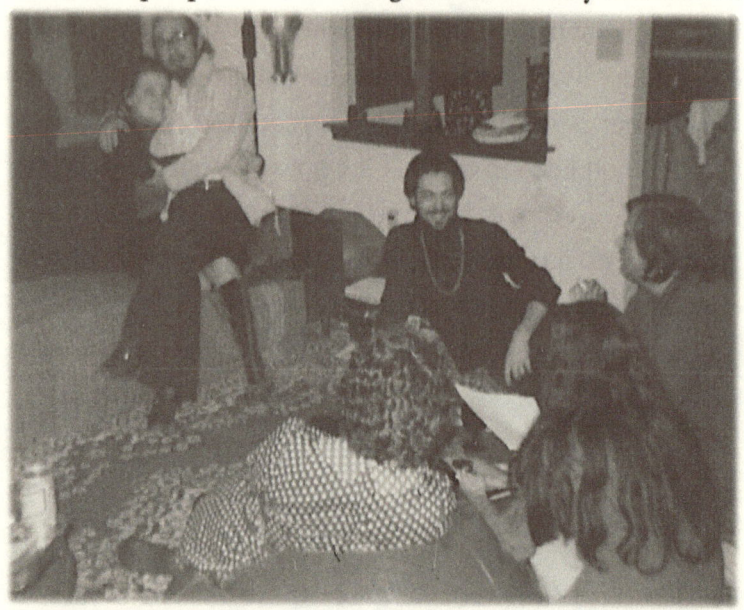

Opera soirée at Teresa's house, with Richard Voinche, stage director

Many good things were happening in our life. Thomas was appointed a magistrate judge of the federal court and was sworn in in Detroit. When we got home, Licia seemed sad. We inquired why, and she said, "Does that mean that when he comes home I have to stand up?" We said nothing would change as far as her dad was concerned. I felt her anguish and promised myself to keep the dialogue open with my Licia. All seemed well, but another storm was brooding over our peaceful existence.

6

An Unexpected New Problem

It was the end of the 1989 school year, and my professional life was booming. I had been appointed the education director of the International School, which was comprised of German, French, Spanish, Italian and American students whose parents were involved with the automobile industry.

The founder of the school was a state senator, Jack Faxon, a real fox, who saw an opportunity to make money and took advantage by making tuition very high, knowing it would be paid by the

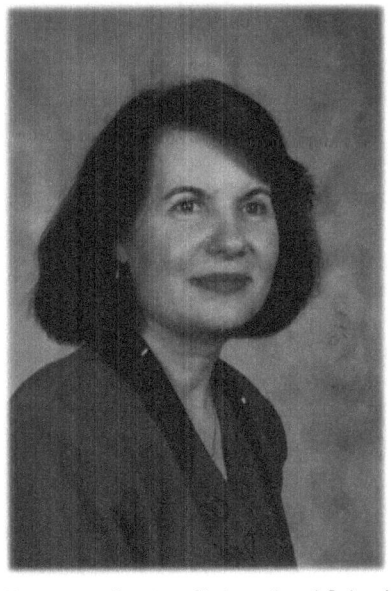
Teresa as director of International School

various companies that employed the families. I wanted the Black students, many from the inner city in Detroit, to also have an opportunity to attend, so the parents and I held many scholarship fundraising events, including concerts thanks to the generosity of my opera singer and teacher, Emilia Cundari. Emilia had a big following, having sung at La Scala and at the Metropolitan in New York. She was made renowned by a book published in Italy, which listed her as one of the fifty best singers of Italy. She and I became very good friends, both of us from Calabria and sharing a love of music.

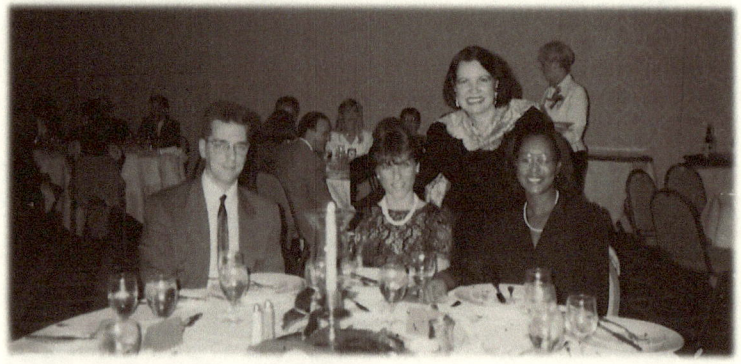

Teresa with parents at an International School benefit concert

One Friday night, a few children had remained at Latch-key, an after-school program. Many were always picked up late, their mothers being professionals, so I understood their dilemma and would often take them home and feed them. That particular evening a father with a four-year-old came into my office and asked the child to stand outside, to which I objected. I took the child back to preschool where the teacher, a Lebanese woman, stressed that the child should not stay in her class. I went back and told the father, who said to me, in a menacing way, that the child WOULD remain at the International School. I tried to explain that with his daughter's speech impediment, regular exposure to another language would be frustrating for her, as the teachers had observed. He informed me that Senator Faxon said that she could stay, and he put his hand in his pocket as if he had a gun. (I knew he was a police officer.) But I told him I had to leave and I left, saying goodbye to the children and the few remaining teachers. I trembled all the way home.

After supper and everyone had gone to bed, I sat at the piano singing a few melodies, hoping that my heart, which was racing like an automobile engine, would calm down. And if singing couldn't do it, nothing would. It didn't help, and I woke Thomas up, telling him I thought I was in the middle of a heart attack and to take me to Beaumont Hospital without delay. We got in the car and sped like maniacs, going through every yellow light. We checked in at the emergency room, where the moment you announce heart attack everything is on speed dial. Dr. Friedman, my cardiologist, was parking his car and I called him to be in the cath lab immediately. It was life and death. I was awake through the whole procedure, a balloon angioplasty, where a balloon was inserted through a catheter from the main artery in my groin to the point of the blockage, and then expanded to remove the blockage. It was a delicate operation because my veins were very small due to the prior radiation and the fact that the catheters were made mostly for men, whose veins are bigger than females'. Everything was successful, however, and my crushing pain disappeared. I was taken to intensive care, where a fifty-pound weight was applied on my groin to prevent any bleeding and to prevent blood cloths from forming, all of which required my body to be immobile for a few days.

A month after the heart attack, Thomas and I went for a walk and suddenly I felt a pain in the inside of my left arm. We went back home and I took some nitro pills, which did not eliminate the pain, and I decided to call an ambulance, which came immediately. In the emergency room, they found my heart enzymes were elevated, and then immediately to the cath lab for another angioplasty, which unplugged the closed vein. Again in the intensive care unit, immobile for two days with the fifty-pound weight on my groin to stop the vein from bleeding. This time our Licia was there with me, and I felt comforted. I returned home a week later, amid a torrent of rain which reminded both Licia and me of *One Hundred Days of Solitude* by Marquez, in which the author described how it rained for one hundred days. It was good to be home and to listen to the rain tumbling steadily from the sky.

The following summer I went for a walk with my

friend Aurelia in the midday sun. On the way back we climbed a hill and I fainted, a fall which fortunately Aurelia broke. Close to home, she walked to my house to fetch her car, leaving me in the hands of the neighbor who came to help. We sat in my garden and we decided it was heat exhaustion. I went to see my cardiologist the next day, but he was on vacation. His assistant examined me and, fortunately, did not identify the event as any cardiac failure.

7

To Europe with a Knapsack

In 1996, my cardiologist mentioned that I was becoming a heart invalid and it was time to do something daring. I took him seriously and left for Switzerland. I met my dear friend Ursula at the airport in Frankfurt, Germany. From there we visited the Philosophers' Trail in the Swiss Alps, in honor of my Licia, who was teaching philosophy, and we stayed in this lovely village for a few days. Then I went to Frankfurt, where I visited several of my students and their families: the Stegers and the Ghoussainis. After a brief visit, Hilary Steger and I left for Prague by train.

At the border between Germany and the Czech Republic, the train personnel changed to Czech. A police officer came on board and asked for passports, and when I showed him my Canadian passport, he announced that all Canadians had to get off the train immediately. Incredulous, I thought that they did not mean Canadians. I looked for my Italian passport but I had left it at home.

Hilary and I got off the train, and with menacing dogs we were escorted into a little dark room, no telephone, or ability to call out. Two ladies who pretended not to speak German, French, English or Italian kept interrogating us in Czech, neither of us speaking the language. Hilary told me later that they were using menacing tones to try to get money from us, but that if we took the bait and offered them a sum that was not to their liking, they would charge us with the crime of trying to bribe them. After a few hours, still guarded by dogs, we boarded the train for Munich. We had a great time there, going to the opera, and sitting in what was once the royal box, thanks to Mr. Steger, Hilary's husband. Hilary later read in the German paper that Canada had asked all the Czech Gypsies to leave the country, hence the retaliation against Canadians traveling to the Czech Republic. A few days later I left for Hungary, another frightening adventure.

I boarded the train to Hungary on a first-class ticket. It seemed that I was the only one in the whole car. The conductor came for my ticket and announced that the amount I paid in the U.S. for the ticket was not sufficient. I replied that I did not travel with money but I would be glad to withdraw from my account in Budapest and pay the due amount. He came by several times giving me intimidating looks, but I tried to remain composed and pretend I did not fear him. After an arduous trip, we arrived in Budapest, where my friend Gyongyi and her husband met me. We went to the ticket office and I informed them in French that the conductor standing beside me tried to swindle more money for my first-class ticket. The lady called the police, who came immediately and took him away.

My friend's husband decided that we should visit the Herend Porcelain Factory. The factory visit was interesting; I bought a little coffee set and then we left. The next morning Gyongyi and I visited the surrounding villages, lots of art displays, and very interesting. I later went to a Marriott Hotel on the banks of the Danube, where the manager gave me a beautiful room overlooking the river. There I met a physician friend with her physicist son, and I invited them to breakfast the next day. They had been reduced to poverty by the communist party when they refused to join it. Communism was felt everywhere you went in the country, notwithstanding the Revolution of 1956.

I met up with Gyongyi later and we had a good time visiting Budapest, a beautiful musical city. A few days later we took the train to Szeged, the city where Gyongyi's family lived. There we stayed with her friend, a judge, and her senator husband, who was in Parliament in Budapest. Her house was lovely, but eerie, with life-size clay statues standing or sitting around. I was spooked. I was still recovering from two heart attacks, but Gyongyi insisted in the middle of the afternoon, under a burning sun, that we walk to a cemetery not too far away. However, we walked for a long time, crossing a bridge. I was exhausted, but she insisted that we were almost there. It was the most daunting trip. Back at the judge's home, Gyongyi decided we should all go to a concert, but no longer trusting her, I declined. No sooner had the others left, that a sweet old lady came in from next door, which was separated from the judge's house by a thick evergreen fence. She had a bottle and two glasses, filled them up and signaled me to drink; leaving shortly afterwards. I later asked Gyongyi who she was, and she said she was the judge's mother, who was still afraid of the communist regime, whose members forced accusatory confessions from family members.

The next day we went to the center of Szeged. We visited Gyongyi's aunt, who was an opera diva and who, accompanied on the piano by her devoted husband, sang a Lehar aria in German. Her frail voice spoke of greater days on the opera stage. She was a sweet lady and her husband adored her, manifested by his pleased face at the end of her singing. It was so good to see two old people still touched by the magic of love. We left after a brief visit, and then went home, packed and left the next morning for Vienna. Music was everywhere, especially from the main street, which was closed to traffic so that people could stroll leisurely among the musicians, who played various instruments. A joyful city. From Vienna we went to Salzburg, a small city whose main piazza was encircled by four walls, each with an arched portico leading out into the city. We visited Mozart's home in a tall apartment in the main wall. We bought tickets to a Mozart performance in a concert hall and then visited an old cemetery with an outdoor beer parlor. We drank beer and ate sandwiches and in the evening we attended the concert, a combination of singing and instrumental music. Then we boarded the train for Italy and crossed the majestic Alps, lighted by the little villages in the valleys at the foot of the towering, majestic mountains. When we entered Italy it was morning, and I felt relieved to see blue sky, although Salzburg and Vienna were culturally vibrant cities bathed in art and history.

Then we went to Verona and visited the house of Romeo and Juliet, which has become a favorite stop for tourists, although they never lived there. From there we visited our friends, Marianna and Gian Franco Del Santo, in Torbole, who lived in a house in the hills with a magnificent view of Lago di Garda. We were treated to a sumptuous supper and then coffee on the balcony, watching the little nearby villages around the lake come to life as their lights came on. The next day we visited some of those medieval villages nestled in the hills with charming, narrow ascending and descending roads, which would tire even the best athlete. We made it down to the city of Torbole and had a great lunch and visited shops. We climbed back to Marianna's place for a *pisolino*. In the evening Gian Franco took us to a famous restaurant for an unforgettable supper, then to a charming cafe where Gyongyi and Gian Franco talked about a Hungarian professor of medicine at the University of Padova. We left for Perugia the next morning, where we met the bass baritone Sergio Pezzetti, who took us to a nearby *agroturismo* for supper in a beautiful farmhouse, a bounteous five-course meal made with fresh food grown on the premises. We ate family style *all'aperto* (in the open) with a splendid view of Perugia, followed by a visit to the city and his studio, where students were waiting for a lesson. What a delight to hear him sing from *Rigoletto* and *The Barber of Seville*, where he really showed his artistry, not only as a singer but also a comic. He had the perfect face, plastic-like, which he could mold easily to fit the characters, a real master of the opera buffa.

The following morning we set out for Assisi, the crown jewel of the region Umbria, where the Church of Saint Francis of Assisi called you to prayer with the holy atmosphere that prevailed. A real medieval marvel, full of frescoes painted by Giotto, father of the Renaissance. We also visited the Lower Church, where Saint Francis's remains supposedly rest in a mausoleum. What remained chiseled in my mind was the fresco depicting Francis, half naked, having taken off his silk clothes and thrown them at his father. A work of art which stands as a masterpiece of colors, forms and details. In subsequent years when I visited Assisi with my family, my Thomas was denied entrance to the church because he was wearing shorts, a decision which Thomas challenged by pointing out that Saint Francis himself was naked, showing more than parts of his legs. But, neither my brilliant lawyer's argument, nor my offer to give a big donation, could persuade the priest to make an exception.

Then we began our descent and visited some of the artisans of the area, working and selling their creations. I bought several items made of copper worked in a unique way typical of the area (copper battuto, chiseled or hammered in a way that left circular indentations on the surface). I still cherish my pieces. We visited silk makers and bought many scarves, which we gave as gifts to my relatives in Capistrano. Enzo, my cousin from Parma, visited us back in Perugia, where we visited the silk factory owned by Saint Francis's father and the balcony above, where Francis was supposedly kept prisoner by his father, who did not approve of his ascetic life. We had an exquisite meal in a restaurant with a cave-like ambience, and we noticed that many customers were sending us drinks and hors d'oeuvres. To our surprise we learned later from the waiter that the people at the restaurant thought I was the singer performing in the piazza that night, so much was my resemblance to her. We proceeded to the piazza and were treated to a concert *all'aperto* with popular melodies and excerpts from operas. I had bought so many items that we had to buy a suitcase to carry them all. Goodbye to my resolution of traveling light with a knapsack.

Early in the morning we took the train to Rome and then south to Calabria, enjoying some of the most inspiring scenery as the train went along the Tyrrhenian coast, with its long white beaches shining under the ever-brilliant sun. At one o'clock in the afternoon, we were treated to another unforgettable meal on the train, served on white tablecloths by waiters in black tuxedos, with wine in abundance in tall crystal glasses. Inebriated, we fell asleep for the customary *pisolino*. We woke up to colorful cannoli served with espresso; what a feast! In the evening we enjoyed a sunset glowing like a ball of fire casting images on the crystalline sea, and then we saw, nestled in a hill, the *terme* (hot baths) quite renowned during the Roman and Greek eras. The train arrived in Pizzo, where a joyful cousin Luigi met us and took us to Capistrano, to his house where another sumptuous meal prepared by Nonna awaited us. We all ate and drank homemade wine. Luigi's three young boys entertained us with school and village life stories, and an enormous plate of fruits was served, including my favorite, figs. What joy to be among people I loved and cherished. The only inconvenience was that I had to translate for my friend, who spoke not a word of Italian, but she was pleasant and joyful, happy to be among loving and generous people.

8

Capistrano, Visiting My Aunts and Gyongyi's Story

The next day we went to visit my aunts. Zia Maria, the nun, now mother to her own children, who first mothered me, invited us to dinner the next day. Then we proceeded toward Zia Albina's house, crossing the bridge under which I came into the world. The river was singing its eternal song, and we stopped to enjoy its murmuring gurgles as it went to join the sea and become one with the universe. I could have stayed there forever, but Zia Albina was waiting in her garden, busy canning tomatoes. Before we joined her, I advised Gyongyi to take off her dangling earrings, for my aunt would go straight to pull her ears as she usually did. There she was, a little woman scarcely five feet tall with Herculean strength, managing bushels of tomatoes by herself. We went into the house, where we had coffee and taralli, donut-like cookies made with the same dough as the *voti* for the Feast of Saint Rocco in

September. Those were the breads shaped as an array of body parts offered to the saint, who was supposed to heal the villagers' malaises. We went back to Luigi's house for another scrumptious meal, fresh fish fried in olive oil, vegetables prepared in a myriad of ways, fresh crusty bread made in the village, wine, fruits and espresso, followed by a *pisolino*. Unable to sleep, I got up, and like a cat, went into the kitchen, where I saw Francesco, a fifteen-year-old, reading Ovid in Latin to his Nonna, who was lying on the couch. I sat and listened to his melodious, warm voice pronouncing every word with precision and the right inflection, as if he were reading in class; a pleasure to listen to Latin when read well. After Francesco had finished, I asked why he would read in Latin, a language unknown to Nonna, to which Francesco responded in Italian: "Zia, la Nonna adora ascoltare la mia voce" (Aunt, Nonna loves to listen to my voice). This boy does not suffer an inferiority complex, I thought; he will go far in life. Which he did, placing first in the nation in the exams to become a federal criminal magistrate. Everyone eventually got up for espresso; what an idyllic life.

Later in the afternoon we met Marianna, Zia Albina's older daughter, who came from Vibo Valentia with her daughter, Valentina, a precocious six-year-old who was knowledgeable in the history of the area. But before we left we decided with Carlo, her youngest brother, to show Gyongyi "Susu," where Aunt Albina had extensive land.

We climbed the hill in a Fiat on curvy, narrow roads flanked by colorful, scented ginestra. It seemed we were climbing the mountain to Paradise.

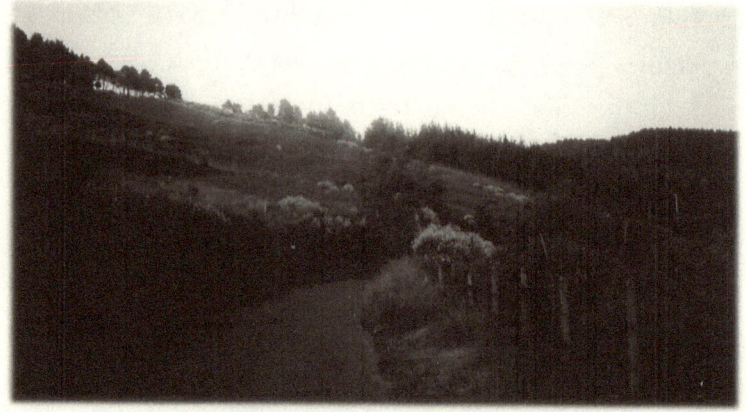

Ginestra adorning the road to Capistrano

There we sat under the majestic pines and listened to the gurgling of the fountain, which offered cold, mineral-laden water, and we drank with pleasure. Marianna and I talked of the trip to Vibo, her work at the museum where she was an archeologist and the artist who would draw in situ the artifacts as they were discovered. She talked about her friend who had bought a piece of property on which to build a house; as they excavated, they found an ancient wall, which necessitated halting construction. The city began excavation and they found a Greek necropolis, a City of the Dead. Not surprising, because this region was part of the Magna Grecia, which extended from Sicily to Campania, the region known for Naples, Pompeii and

Paestum. We all got in the Fiat and descended to Capistrano, where we had coffee; then we left for Marianna's house in Vibo, a Spanish city built on a promontory which offered a splendid view of the Mediterranean Sea.

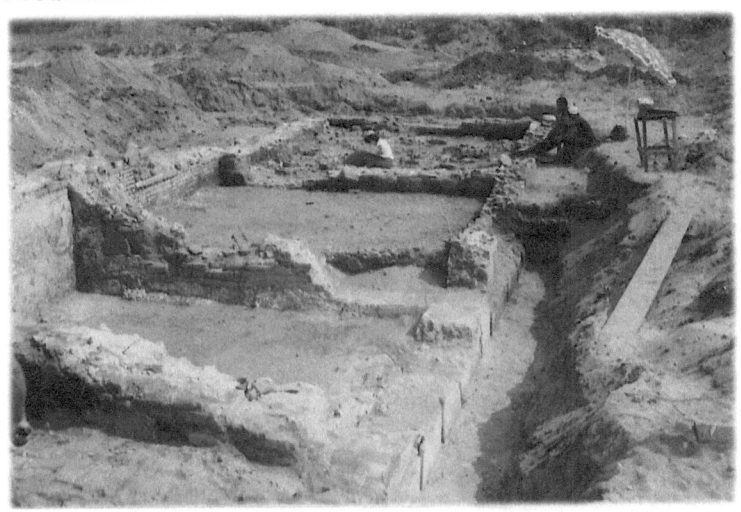

Marianna at the excavation of the necropolis, Vibo Valentia

At the museum we saw the pre-Hellenic vase Marianna had discovered in the sarcophagus of a child, a small, perfect vase, with designs of the underworld on beige ceramic with black borders. It was a model of perfection and harmony of shapes and colors, a treat for the eye; and to think that my Marianna had held it in her hands when it was removed, with a net under her hands to safeguard against dropping it on the ground. Valentina took it all in and then, bored, went to the excavation where her mother followed her, telling her to stop dancing on the site for it was sacred ground. We went to a gelateria for ice cream and then decided to go to Vibo Marina for dinner. Marianna's husband, also an artist working with the city, joined us. We ate al fresco, under a pergola (grapevine) right on the sea, listening to the gentle coming and going of the waves as they kissed the shore. All seemed surrealistic, a corner of the world where life was celebrated and lived to the fullest.

Marianna, a great guide whose love for Calabria shines through her eyes, took us to Tropea, a small city situated on a promontory and extending into the sea, with pristine beaches whose white, powdery sand glistens under the rays of the ever-shining sun. What an enchanted place!

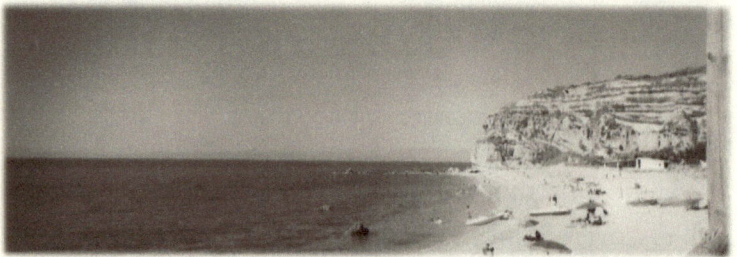

Tropea

We walked on the beach, our bare feet caressing the sand until it felt like white fire, prompting us to find refuge under an umbrella at a cafe, situated on a promontory overlooking the ever-present sea, for a light lunch.

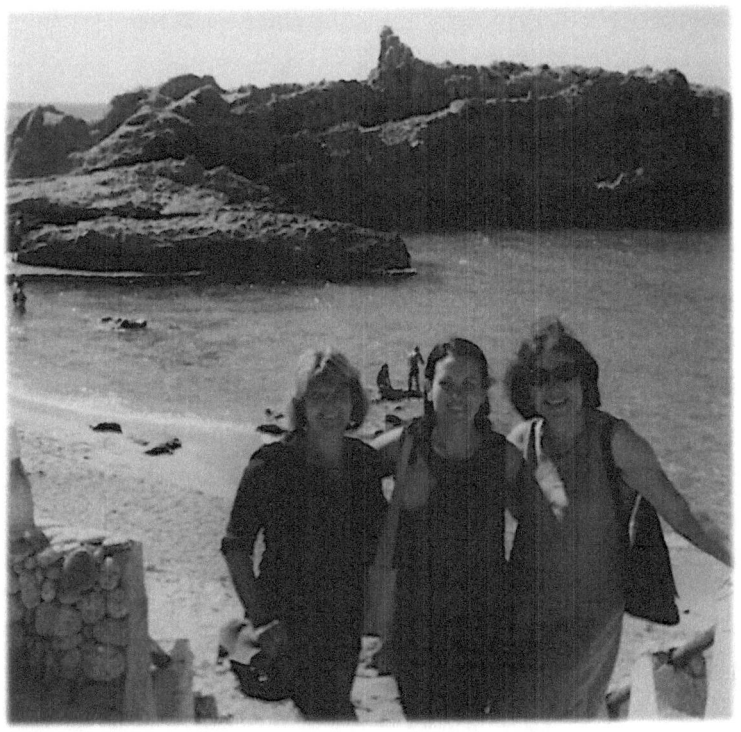

Gyongyi, Marianna and Teresa in Tropea

Marianna told us about her new project at the museum investigating the ancient Mulini a Vento (windmills), which were numerous through Calabria. They were monitored fiercely during World War II by Mussolini Blackshirts to assure that all the flour went to feed the soldiers, often leaving the inhabitants of the village to starve. We devoured our lunch and topped it off with a gelato, the best in the region. In the evening we returned to Capistrano, our last evening with Luigi's family, and then left for Rome early the following morning.

On the train we reminisced about our trip over a continental breakfast, followed by the sumptuous one o'clock dinner served with soave wine. What a voyage I had with my friend, a voyage planned when we first met as students at Harbord Collegiate in Toronto in 1958. In Rome we were met by more cousins; Gyongyi left for Hungary and I went to visit with the Renda side of the family. Gyongyi was taken with Italy, especially Calabria, where we stayed with cousin Luigi and his family. Gyongyi later wrote her recollections of the trip and about her love for Italy, especially Calabria. I share some of them with the reader now:

"Dear Teresa, my best friend, my soul mate. My first introduction to Italy was through Michelangelo, from a book about the Sistine Chapel which I received in 1956 from my parents. I have always loved books but this was special, page after page about the ceiling, still in its faded, pastel condition and that's the way I have always loved it. I could not believe something so unbelievably wonderful could exist on earth. I met my Teresa in high school at Harbord Collegiate, and she became my closest friend for life. She happened to be Italian. It gave me the chance to connect with her Italian family. How can one really connect with Italy unless one connects with an Italian family first?

"I travelled extensively through Italy and thought I

really knew the country, but the knowledge of how little I knew came when Teresa and I entered Italy by train. Teresa is fully alive in everything she does, and I am used to her exuberance, but the moment we entered Italy and saw the red tile roofs, it was as if a volcano erupted. The hills, the flowers, the buildings took on a special significance; the sun infused them with a special light. It was as if the country was glowing, was lifted above ground to eye level, to be felt and seen more closely, to be touched and smelled, and we hadn't even arrived in Calabria at the tip of the boot. Where Teresa was born is where I discovered where the cradle of Italy really is. The cradle of the Roman Empire must have come from there where the Greeks touched first before Rome became the chosen city.

"Teresa's cousin Luigi came to meet us at the train station, driving us to the village through the winding road, with tall grass on either side, getting to know the land moment by moment, when we could see through the grass. Finally we arrived in Capistrano, driven there by a driver who knew every curve in the road, and took each with knowledge, love and assurance. The earth itself came alive as if we were following a well-known path within the human body. Then Capistrano revealed itself, where the swallows had touched down in their flight; Oh! how I loved that place and I hadn't even been introduced to the people of the town; that took place in the days that followed. Luigi's family was comprised of his wife, Rosanna, three boys and grandmother, Teresa, who lived with them and took care of the household. We all sat at the family table where I tasted the product of the land: zucchini flowers coated with a mixture of egg, flour and water and fried to perfection, and many other great dishes, *risotto al frutti di mare,* salads, fruits etc.

"On our first walk in town, heading to the church, we were stopped so many times by family members that I finally asked Teresa, is there anyone here you are not related to? She laughed and said, wait until we visit my aunt

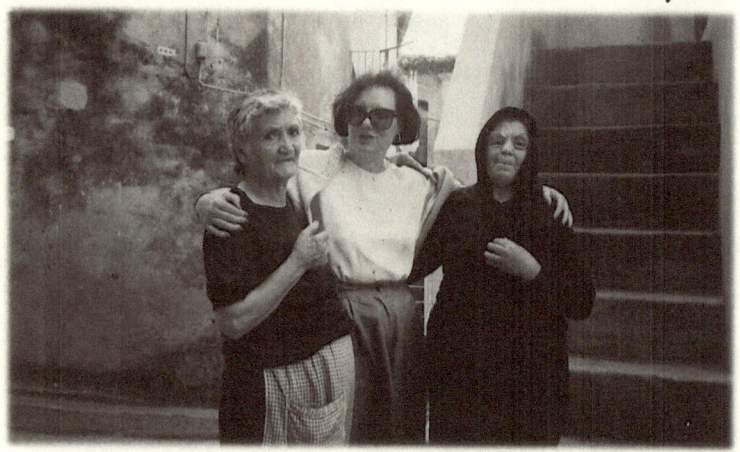
Teresa with women of Capistrano

Albina; make sure you don't wear any earrings, she likes to pull your earlobes in her excitement. I remember the church, where one can drop in anytime of the day for prayer, for peace and quiet, where family history was present at every corner; the frescoes, one on each side of the Baptistry, supposedly painted by Renoir as a gift to the village that gave him hospitality; the house where Teresa was born; the archway where she played hide-and-seek, the olive groves that belonged to her family; the cemetery where her ancestors were buried. The family history began to unravel; the Greeks on her mother's side, her paternal grandmother emigrating from a small town outside Mantova to Brazil, marrying her Calabrese beloved, and coming back to Capistrano; the grandmother cultured, well travelled and wise, educating the village children. The village people lived through special events; the war, finding refuge near a monastery where monks seldom spoke. When it was time to celebrate, the blossoms had to be collected; when someone was ill, family members and villagers sat by the bedside. Birth, death, illness, were no secret to anyone; they were part of their daily lives, nothing hidden away and sterilized. All these experiences were a preparation for life wherever on earth one might find oneself.

"Our friendship has a history, having known each other's parents, with your father calling me Signorina Ginger and giving me bread and wine; my father reciting Italian poetry each time you came. Our lives have evolved, but we have remained connected. You said many years ago: 'One day you have to come where I was born,' and now, forty years later, we have done it."

I never forgot the day we separated in Rome after being together for about a month. How many memories: our visit to Vibo Valentia, the museum and the excavations my cousin Marianna was involved with, our lovely trip to Tropea with Marianna, eating al fresco, the sea with its crystalline purity almost touching our feet, our lively discussion with Marianna about the excavation and the excitement she felt when they opened the sarcophagus of a child and found a small vase of Hellenic origin, how she trembled when she held it for the first time. They had discovered a Greek necropolis. A goodbye to my dear Gyongyi at the train, and I, with my two colossal cousins, proceeded to my late uncle Domenico's house. I missed his buoyant, wide smile, showing his white teeth, but I was glad to see the rest of the family.

My Zia Giuseppina, old but still sharp, recounted a visit to Rome by an old friend, Austin, who had come to Italy in 1967 to propose to me, and with whom she spoke English. How proud she was to remember the English she learned in the U.S. as a child before moving to San Nicola, a village five kilometers from Capistrano. It was good to see this dear old aunt so loved by her numerous family members.

And it transported me back to the end of my visit to Italy in 1967, shortly after I had first met Thomas. It had been a good trip but I was anxious to hear my Thomas's voice on the phone. Soon after my return home, he had a few days off from the army, and decided to come to Toronto, bringing me a beautiful diamond, cut by an artisan in Louisville in the form of a tear. It was beautiful and he gave it to me after a Calabrese dinner my mother had prepared for the occasion, which my beloved Angela, already eight years old, attended, not too happy, for she did not want to see me go to another country. We made tentative plans for our wedding, which was to take place on July 13,1968, at the Newman Chapel at the University of Toronto, with Father Marcel, a friend, officiating.

9

Trip to Montreal Before My Wedding

I wanted to take a trip with my beloved Gina, who was a year older than I, almost a twin, whom I was sorry to leave, and decided to take her to Montreal to visit our sister Pina.

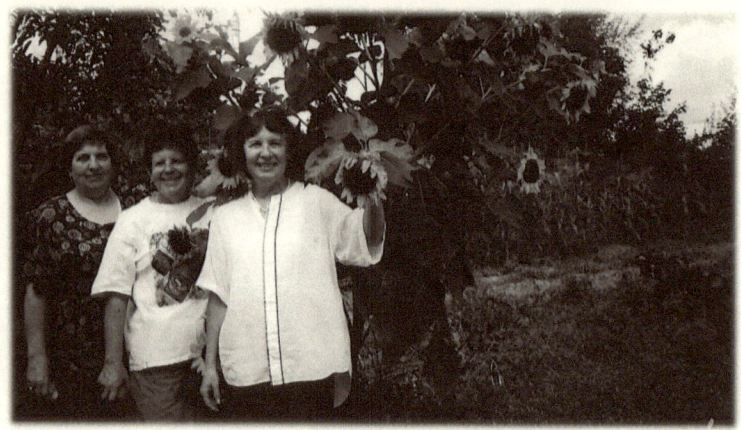

Gina, Pina and Teresa on farm in Montreal

Pina was happy to see us, her little sisters, for whom she had made beautiful silk dresses whose borders she adorned with embroidered flowers. Gina and I had five hours of train ride to reminisce about our childhood back in Capistrano. How happy we were then, notwithstanding the hardships the war imposed on us. She recalled how clean Pina was and how every night she would inspect Gina's feet to see if they were clean enough for Gina to share the bed with her. Most of the time Gina's feet did not meet Pina's standards of cleanliness, and she would drag her to the fountain behind our house to wash her in cold running water. Poor Gina, she kicked and screamed to no avail, with me following them, holding Gina's hand and crying too, for I felt her pain.

It was noon and Gina opened her bag full of delicious food and we began to eat. How thoughtful she was, bringing all the foods I liked, including cherries, my favorite fruit. Then we took a *pisolino* and woke up in the Montreal train station, where Pina and Toto, her husband, came to meet us. At her house we were treated to a delicious supper and planned to visit her farm the next day. I loved Pina's children. They all came to the farm with us and gave us a tour, a paradise of beautiful flowers, plants of every kind bearing fruit, and a pergola (grapevine) in front of the house which Joe, my favorite nephew, told us was built by his parents. The sunflowers dominated the place with their bright yellow corolla and long stems. A beautiful mulberry tree laden with fruits stood erect as a sentinel by the house. It brought back memories of going to gather leaves for the silkworms that we raised for the threads to make cloth for our clothing and other items needed in daily life.

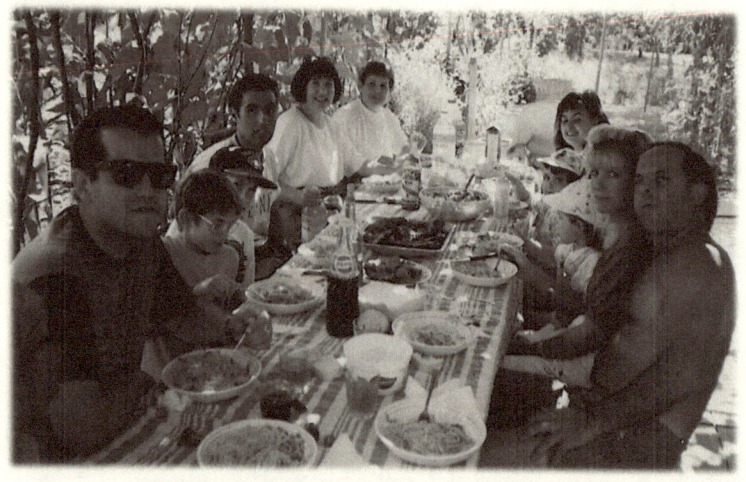
Teresa with Pina and family on farm in Montreal

The next day, bright and early, the farmer next to Pina's farm came to bring milk in huge vats for Pina to make cheese and ricotta, a fascinating process involving several steps: First, bring the milk to almost boiling, then add the rennet to coagulate the milk, which took several hours. The rennet was taken from the inside of the stomach of a newborn goat, which was hung out to dry, and then used to make cheese.

Second, gather the coagulated milk in your hands and put it in forms made of wicker and let it dry totally.

Third, turn the forms upside down and begin the curing process by salting the cheese generously.

TRIP TO MONTREAL BEFORE MY WEDDING

Fourth, put the forms of cheese on a cloth and let them dry until hard.

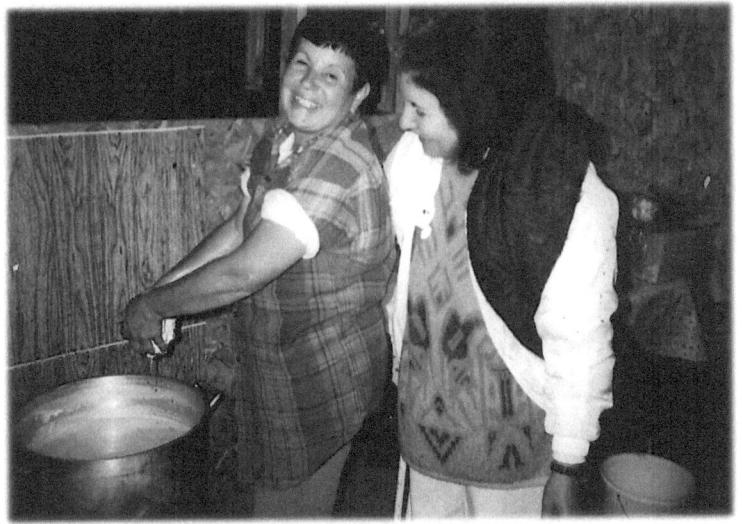

Pina and Teresa, making mozzarella in Montreal

Pina served the cheese she had made the previous year, which was delicious. With the serum left in the pot, add milk and a little vinegar and heat the mixture, stirring it constantly with a long wooden spoon until the ricotta cheese comes to the top, ready to be spooned out. The serum is delicious to drink while it is hot. Gina and I had a great time watching our Pina, who had become a great farmer, an incredible evolution from the village girl who never went to cultivate or gather any produce, and spent her whole day embroidering beautiful flowers and designs on tablecloths, pillowcases and sheets for our dowry. What a transformation!

We left the farm and visited old Montreal, with its majestic Cathedral of Notre Dame, followed by a French lunch. We then visited Saint Joseph's Oratory, with its majestic and steep steps, leading us to the inside of the church, at the center of which was a statue of Saint Joseph with hundreds of crutches around it left by people who had been cured of their infirmities. We prayed and then went to buy souvenirs to bring home as gifts. Toto was very patient in chauffeuring us around and very warm with us. The next day we took the train back to Toronto, where I had to finish preparations for our wedding. Gina was sad to see me go to another country, and she expressed it so touchingly that we both cried. We promised each other that we would stay in touch and that nothing would keep us apart.

To break the tears we talked about our Pina telling us how she defended herself in court in a lawsuit brought by the neighbors for her having built a house on property zoned only as farmland. Our Pina represented herself in front of the judge, telling him that they did have a farm there with crops and animals, but needed a house if it rained and a kitchen with a stove to make their espresso. In addition, their residence in Montreal was quite far from the farm, and they had to cross a long bridge over the Saint Lawrence, which was dangerous at night, especially for two people getting on in years. The judge was so impressed by her arguments, delivered in perfect French, that he dismissed the case. We were so proud of our Pina. What a marvelous trip with my adorable Gina, discovering how our Pina had evolved over the years. Back in Toronto, Thomas was waiting for us and I was happy to see him and to have him help me with the last details of the wedding.

Our wedding was a great success. We had people from many different countries attend, a true international gathering at the Newman Chapel on the campus of the University of Toronto (UT), followed by an elegant reception at Inn on the Park, which offered beautiful grounds and an exquisite classical dining room served by French waiters. A quartet provided by the students of the UT accompanied the meal with delightful pieces. Dancing followed the dinner, to the merriment of many. A wedding to remember! Our honeymoon took us to the Expo 67 grounds in Montreal, where we met, then to New York, where we attended a performance of the ballet *Swan Lake*, followed by an elegant dinner at Biffi's restaurant, where the food was exquisite and the atmosphere classy. The following morning we left for Kentucky, where Thomas was serving his two years of military duty. My mother and his parents visited later, with Thomas's brothers, Wayne and Bruce, and we were delighted to see them and host them in our little abode in Elizabethtown, not too far from Fort Knox. The Vietnam War was raging, and everybody available was being sent there to fight the Viet Cong. I became a teacher of English at the

Army Education Center for returnee soldiers and those who would be sent to combat in the near future. I was saddened by the stories of killing by the returnees and by the fears displayed by those who would have to face combat.

Every day the soldiers would write a short essay on their experiences, 150 pieces of writing per day. Unfortunately, I did not save any of them, although every story still lingers in my memory. My employment did not last long. The captain in charge lacked a sense of humor, which was displayed in my firing for inability to keep order. The students found pleasure in going to the blackboard and writing sentences to be analyzed by the class. One of the sentences was: "Madame Carlson's legs are very beautiful," at which everyone began to laugh. The captain happened to be passing by and, hearing the laughter, came in angrily ordering the students to sit down, and left the classroom. A few minutes later he came back holding a hammer, nails and a piece of cardboard which he nailed to the front of the desk to hide the opening. He called me into the hall and told me I was fired. The students felt badly for me and I was not given a chance to talk with the soldiers and reassure them that it was not their fault. I walked to the JAG office where my husband was working, and told the people there what had happened. My husband explained to me that if I were an American soldier, I would have been tried for insubordination for having told the captain off. But I was glad I was a proud Canadian and remained such until Senator Hilary Clinton ran for president. As a woman, that was one of my prerequisites, the other being an African American candidate. And I did become an American citizen when President Obama was elected. I had the pleasure of having a little ceremony at home (I was in a wheelchair at the time), where one of the immigration officers and my husband swore me in. Our Iranian neighbors, Afsaneh and her children Ala and Ali attended.

Our stay in the army neared its end, and in autumn 1969 we left for Lansing, Michigan. A year later our precious Licia was born, an enchanted child who brought us immense joy all through our life and still continues in spite of my numerous health threats. We all travelled together to my Capistrano the summer of 2018, when I was able to share with my thirteen-year-old grandson, Julian, the places I loved as a child. The young men who attended a party I had thrown in 1967 in the big garden of Maestro Orlando's, music teacher to many of us who were now very accomplished, came to visit me on my cousin Luigi's balcony and still remembered the party we had. It was the first of its kind, just for young people, dancing, playing instruments, eating, and drinking their first punch with the whisky that I had brought from Canada. My Julian was amazed at how many people still cherished and remembered the party and me.

IN MY MISFORTUNE, I AM MOST FORTUNATE

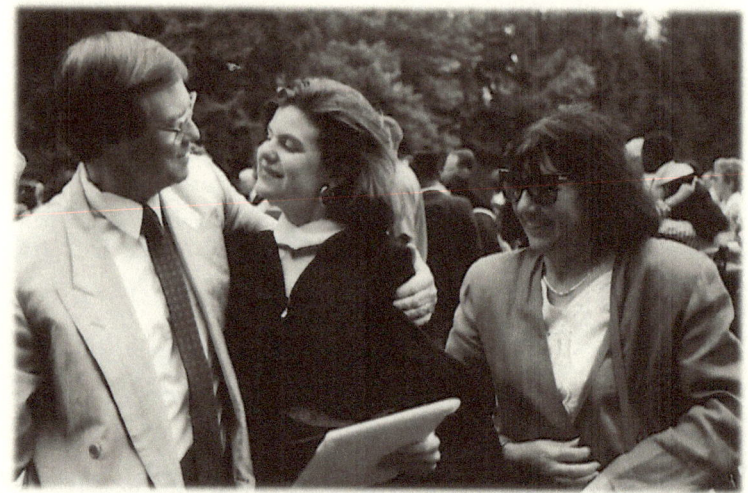

Tom, Licia and Teresa at Licia's college graduation from Vassar

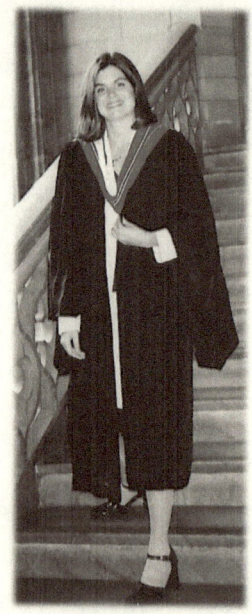

Licia receiving PhD

I have been and continue to be fortunate in my misfortunes. I have enjoyed watching my Licia grow, graduate from college with a PhD in philosophy from the University of Toronto, marry a wonderful doctor, Jeremiah Frank, and was most fortunate to witness the birth of my grandchild, Julian, in Boston. What a blessing, surviving cancer for half a century. In Boston I had a valve replacement using a new method, TAVR (a minimally invasive procedure where a new valve is inserted into the heart without removing the old diseased one), which I qualified for due to my radical mastectomies (too much scar tissue built on the chest for open heart surgery). Another example of misfortune creating fortune.

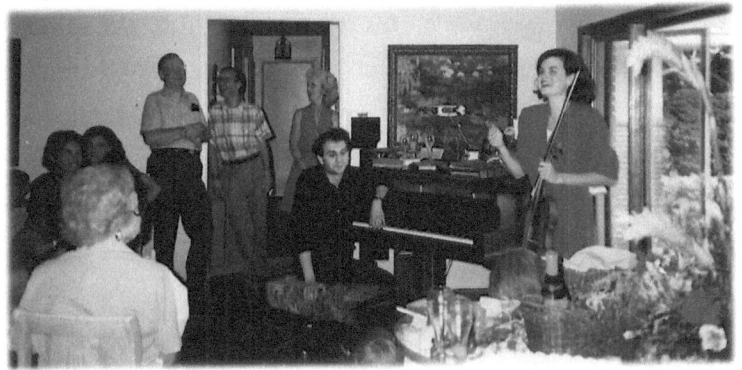

Licia at surprise 50th birthday party for Teresa and Tom in Detroit

On September 1, 2020, we celebrated our Licia's fiftieth birthday, to the delight of us all, many of whom doubted I would see her attend kindergarten, much less a birthday a half century later, due to the terrible prognosis of my breast cancer.

I count my blessings every day and thank God for my transformation into a more sensitive, more altruistic and wiser being, in discerning that which is important from that which is not. This can be difficult at times, but Epictetus, the first-century Greek philosopher who lived in Rome, suggested a solution that requires dividing all things that affect us into those we can control and those we cannot. Thus, we should try to turn our misfortunes into fortunes if we can. There is no cure for cancer, but we can lighten its destructive course by bringing out our better selves and using coping mechanisms that other survivors have used to transform their lives. Above all, we can be positive and, like John Milton says in *Paradise Lost*, turn hell into heaven. As my Nonno Luigi, in simpler parlance, said, we are the puppets and the puppeteer; we can pull the strings of despair or those of strength and survival.

Yes, we can turn our MISFORTUNES into FORTUNES, and I am living proof of it.

www.ingramcontent.com/pod-product-compliance
Lightning Source LLC
Chambersburg PA
CBHW030455010526
44118CB00011B/957